The Diary of a Kitchen

a collection of recipes

Table of Contents

Table of Contents

Table of Contents

Table of Contents

Preparation time: Cook time: Servings:

Ingredients

Method

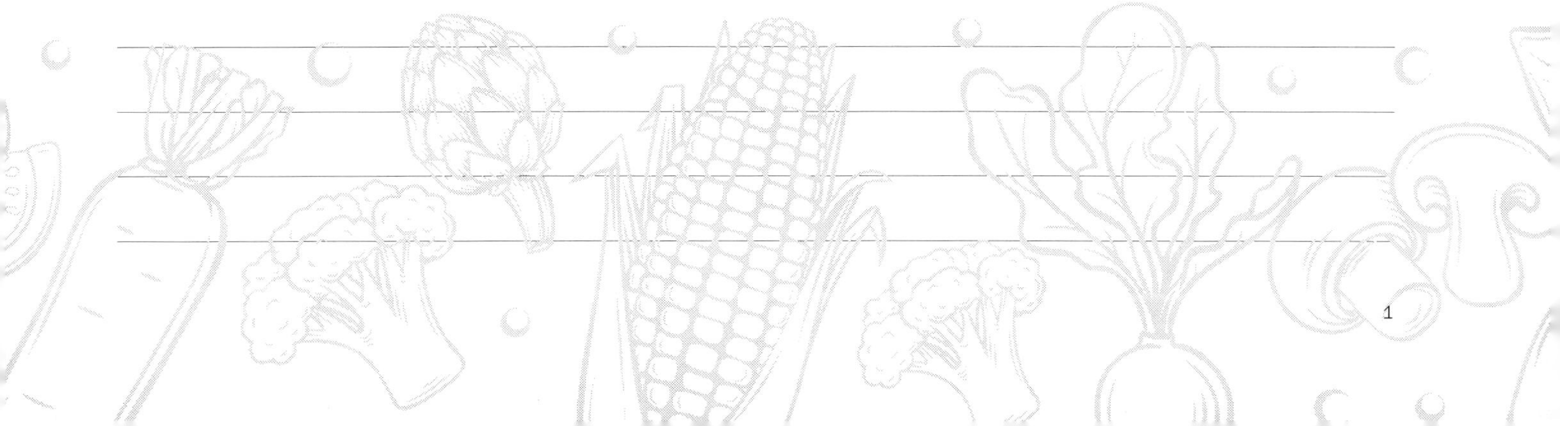

Preparation time: Cook time: Servings:

Ingredients

Method

Preparation time: Cook time: Servings:

Ingredients

Method

Preparation time: Cook time: Servings:

Ingredients

Method

Preparation time: Cook time: Servings:

Ingredients

Method

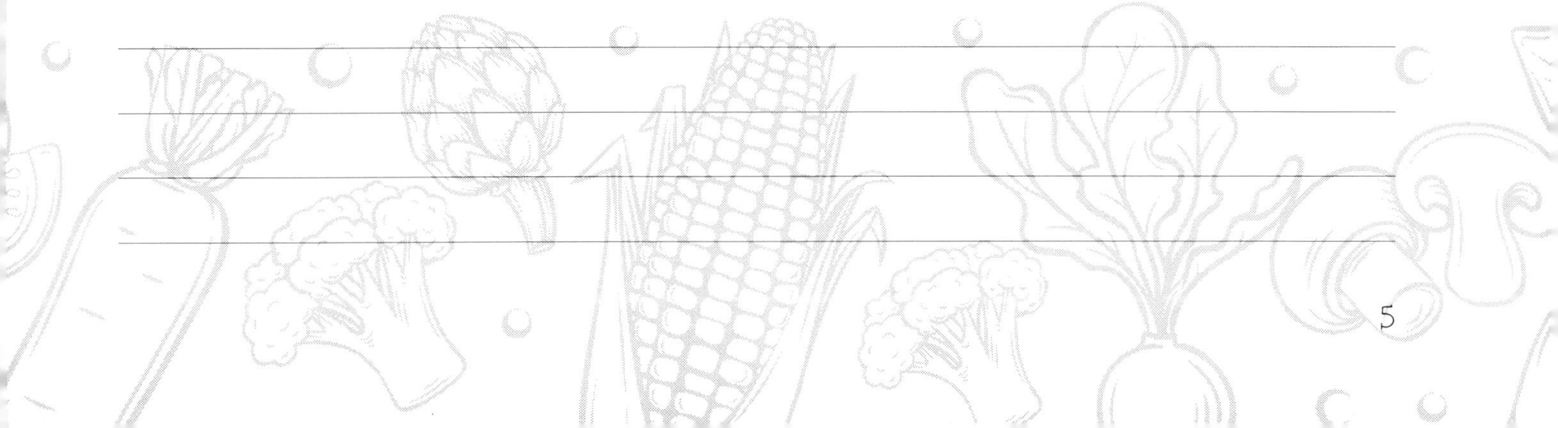

Preparation time: Cook time: Servings:

Ingredients

Method

Preparation time: Cook time: Servings:

Ingredients

Method

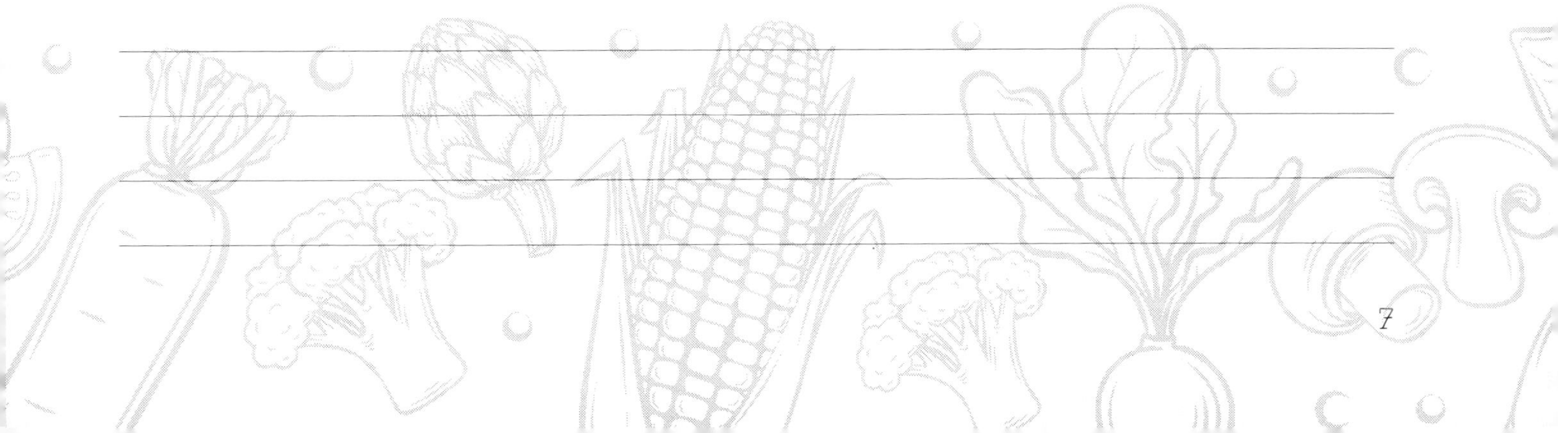

Preparation time: Cook time: Servings:

Ingredients

Method

Preparation time: Cook time: Servings:

Ingredients

Method

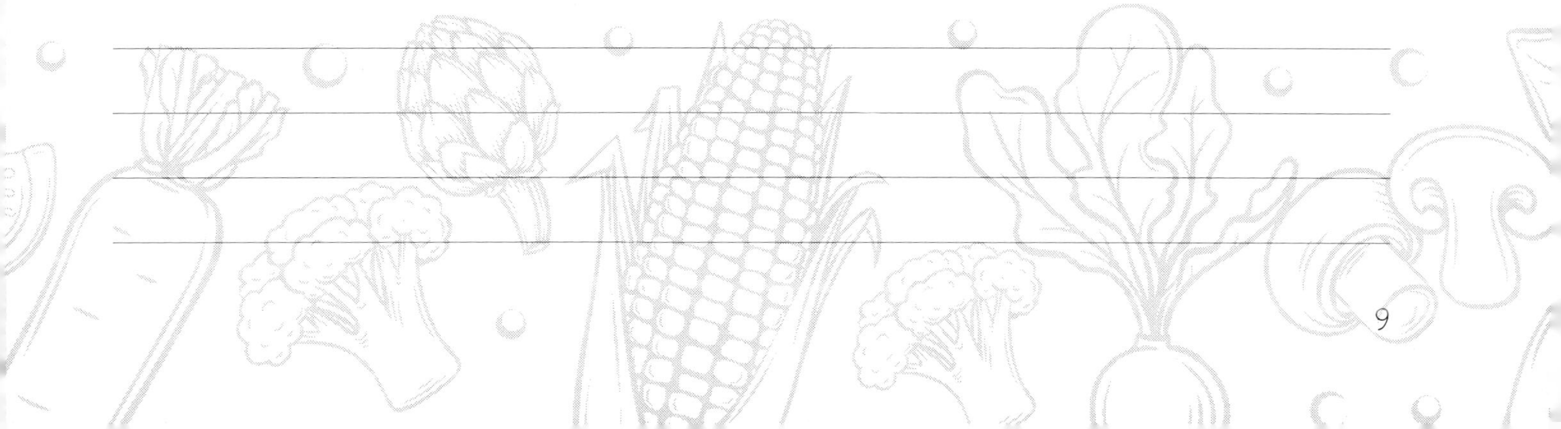

Preparation time: Cook time: Servings:

Ingredients

Method

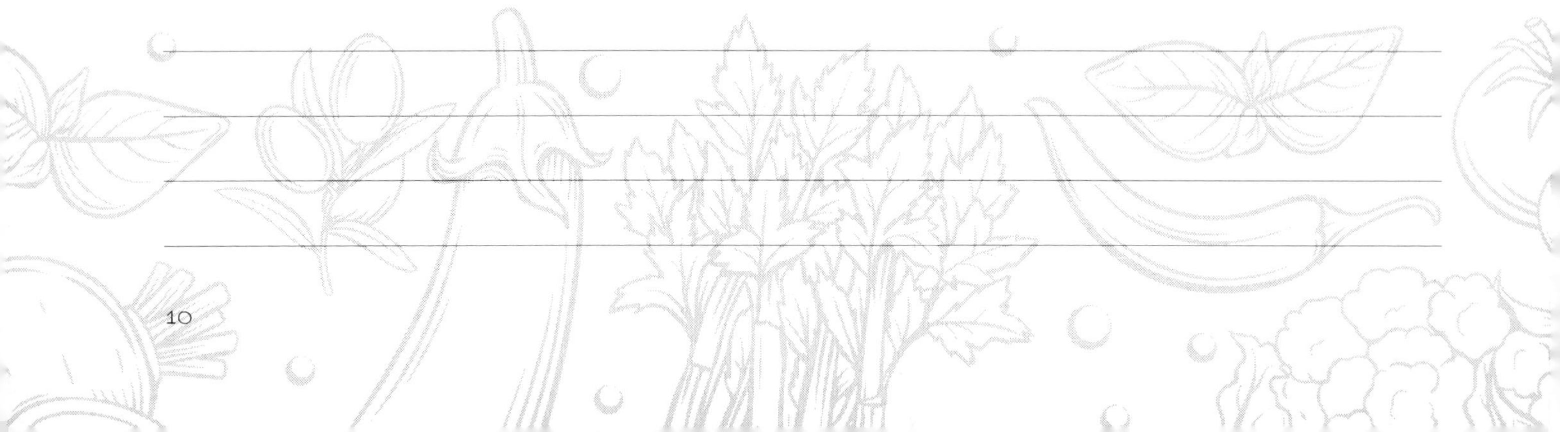

Preparation time: Cook time: Servings:

Ingredients

Method

Preparation time: Cook time: Servings:

Ingredients

Method

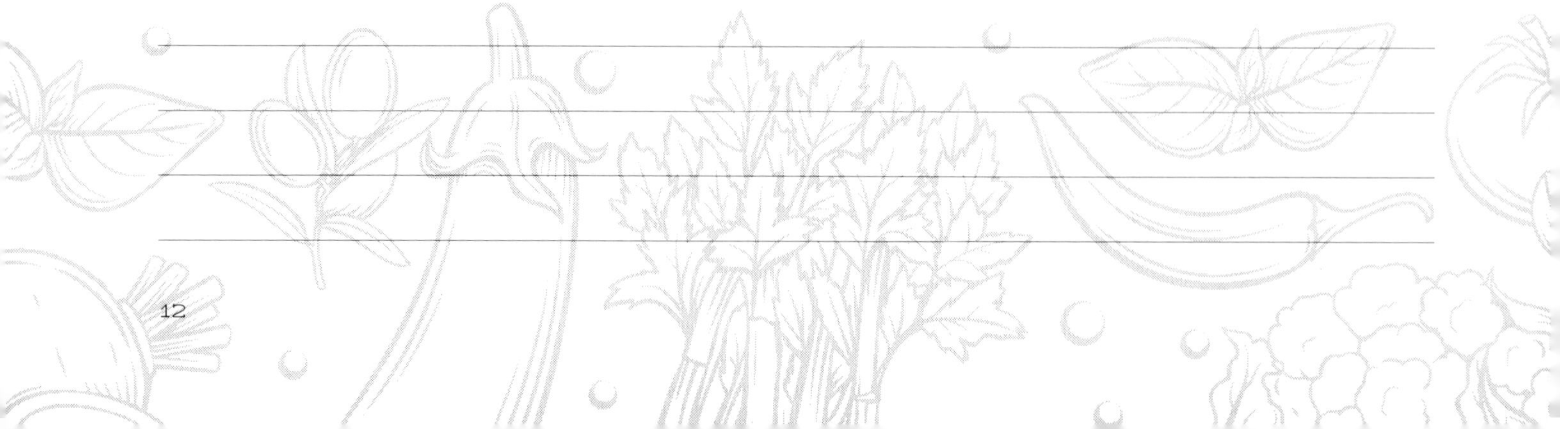

Preparation time: Cook time: Servings:

Ingredients

Method

Preparation time: Cook time: Servings:

Ingredients

Method

Preparation time: Cook time: Servings:

Ingredients

Method

Preparation time: Cook time: Servings:

Ingredients

Method

Preparation time: Cook time: Servings:

Ingredients

Method

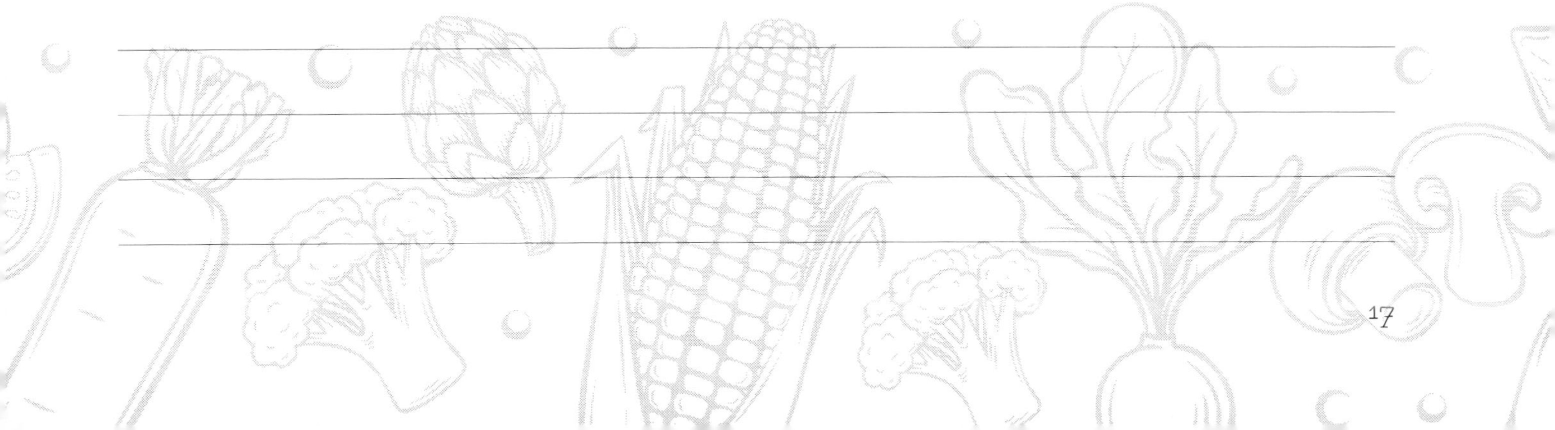

Preparation time: Cook time: Servings:

Ingredients

Method

Preparation time: Cook time: Servings:

Ingredients

Method

Preparation time: Cook time: Servings:

Ingredients

Method

Preparation time: Cook time: Servings:

Ingredients

Method

Preparation time: Cook time: Servings:

Ingredients

Method

Preparation time: Cook time: Servings:

Ingredients

Method

Preparation time: Cook time: Servings:

Ingredients

Method

Preparation time: Cook time: Servings:

Ingredients

Method

Preparation time: Cook time: Servings:

Ingredients

Method

Preparation time: Cook time: Servings:

Ingredients

Method

Preparation time: Cook time: Servings:

Ingredients

Method

Preparation time: Cook time: Servings:

Ingredients

Method

Preparation time: Cook time: Servings:

Ingredients

Method

Preparation time: Cook time: Servings:

Ingredients

Method

Preparation time: Cook time: Servings:

Ingredients

Method

Preparation time: Cook time: Servings:

Ingredients

Method

Preparation time: Cook time: Servings:

Ingredients

Method

Preparation time: Cook time: Servings:

Ingredients

Method

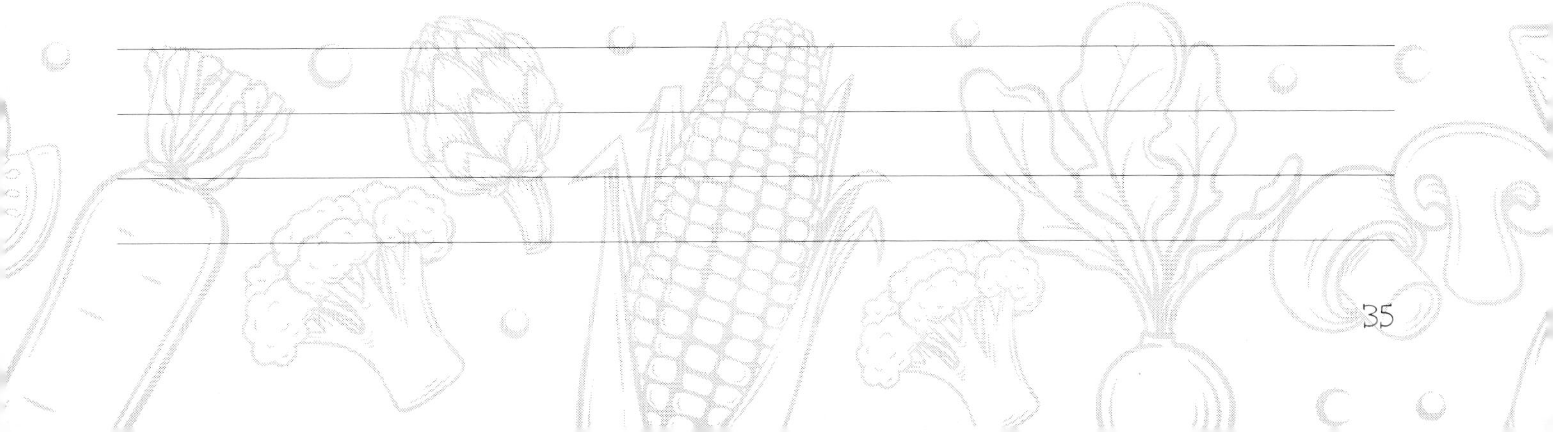

Preparation time: Cook time: Servings:

Ingredients

Method

Preparation time: Cook time: Servings:

Ingredients

Method

Preparation time: Cook time: Servings:

Ingredients

Method

Preparation time: Cook time: Servings:

Ingredients

Method

Preparation time: Cook time: Servings:

Ingredients

Method

Preparation time: Cook time: Servings:

Ingredients

Method

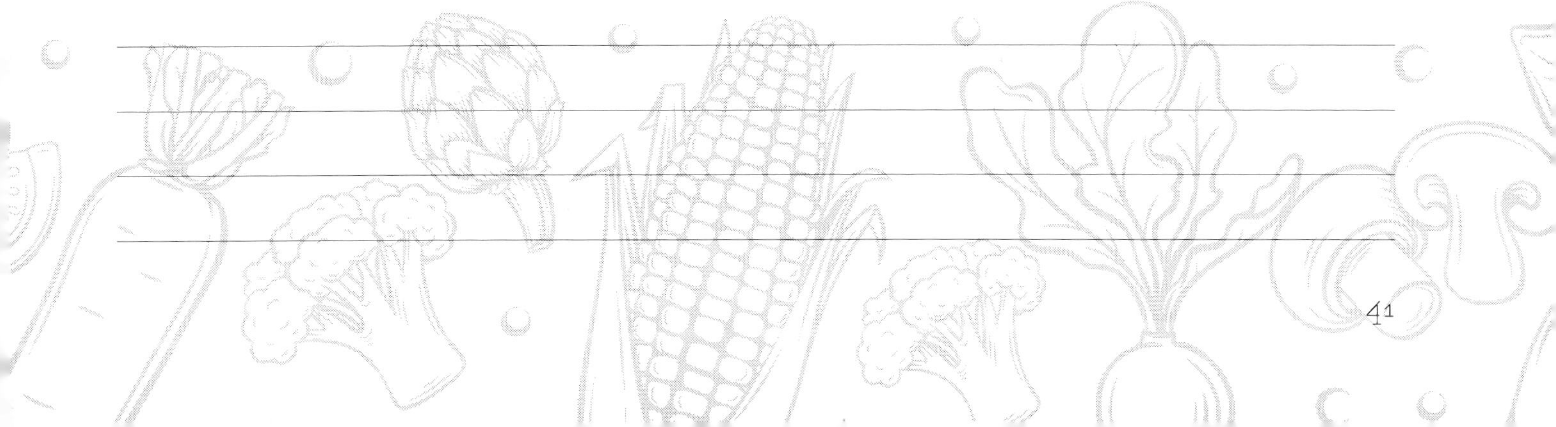

Preparation time: Cook time: Servings:

Ingredients

Method

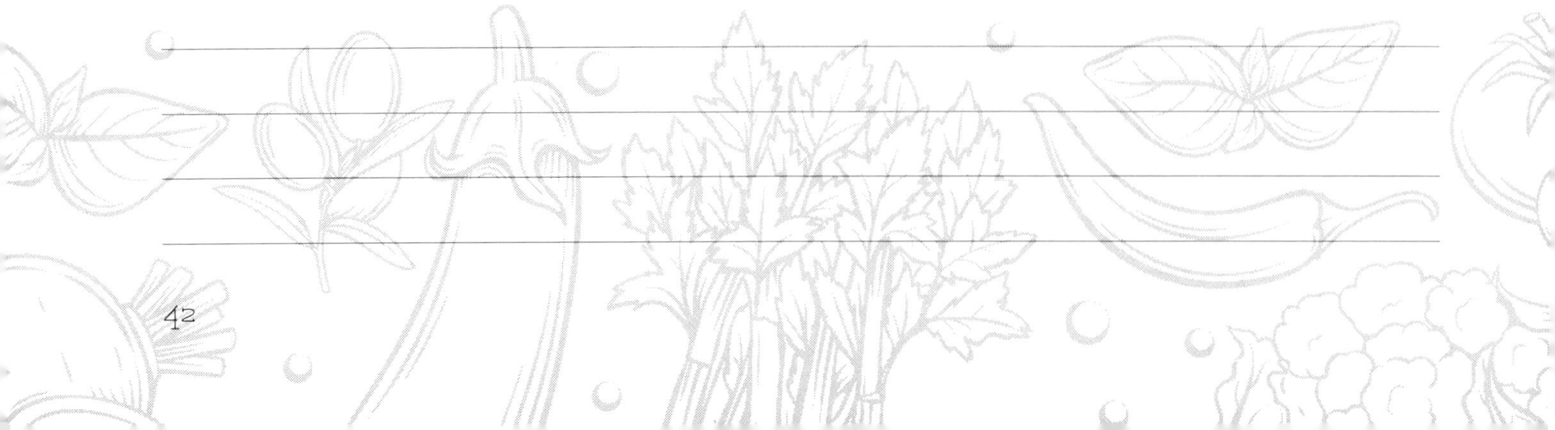

Preparation time: Cook time: Servings:

Ingredients

Method

Preparation time: Cook time: Servings:

Ingredients

Method

Preparation time: Cook time: Servings:

Ingredients

Method

Preparation time: Cook time: Servings:

Ingredients

Method

Preparation time: Cook time: Servings:

Ingredients

Method

Preparation time: Cook time: Servings:

Ingredients

Method

Preparation time: Cook time: Servings:

Ingredients

Method

Preparation time: Cook time: Servings:

Ingredients

Method

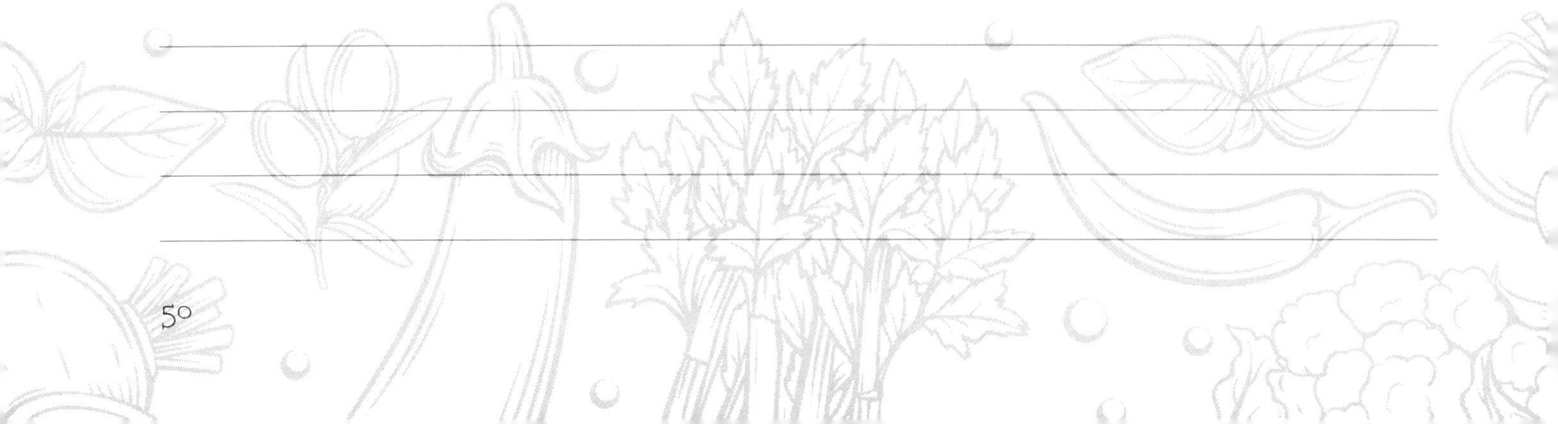

Preparation time: Cook time: Servings:

Ingredients

Method

Preparation time: Cook time: Servings:

Ingredients

Method

Preparation time: Cook time: Servings:

Ingredients

Method

Preparation time: Cook time: Servings:

Ingredients

Method

Preparation time: Cook time: Servings:

Ingredients

Method

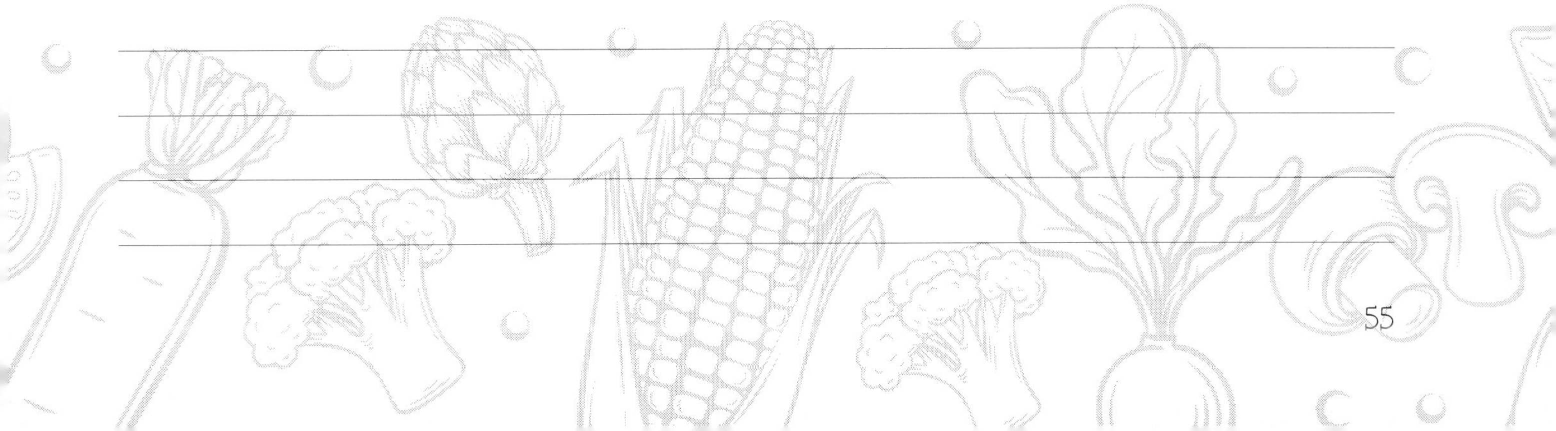

Preparation time: Cook time: Servings:

Ingredients

Method

Preparation time: Cook time: Servings:

Ingredients

Method

Preparation time: Cook time: Servings:

Ingredients

Method

Preparation time: Cook time: Servings:

Ingredients

Method

Preparation time: Cook time: Servings:

Ingredients

Method

Preparation time: Cook time: Servings:

Ingredients

Method

Preparation time: Cook time: Servings:

Ingredients

Method

Preparation time: Cook time: Servings:

Ingredients

Method

Preparation time: Cook time: Servings:

Ingredients

Method

Preparation time: Cook time: Servings:

Ingredients

Method

Preparation time: Cook time: Servings:

Ingredients

Method

Preparation time: Cook time: Servings:

Ingredients

Method

Preparation time: Cook time: Servings:

Ingredients

Method

Preparation time: Cook time: Servings:

Ingredients

Method

Preparation time: Cook time: Servings:

Ingredients

Method

Preparation time: Cook time: Servings:

Ingredients

Method

Preparation time: Cook time: Servings:

Ingredients

Method

Preparation time: Cook time: Servings:

Ingredients

Method

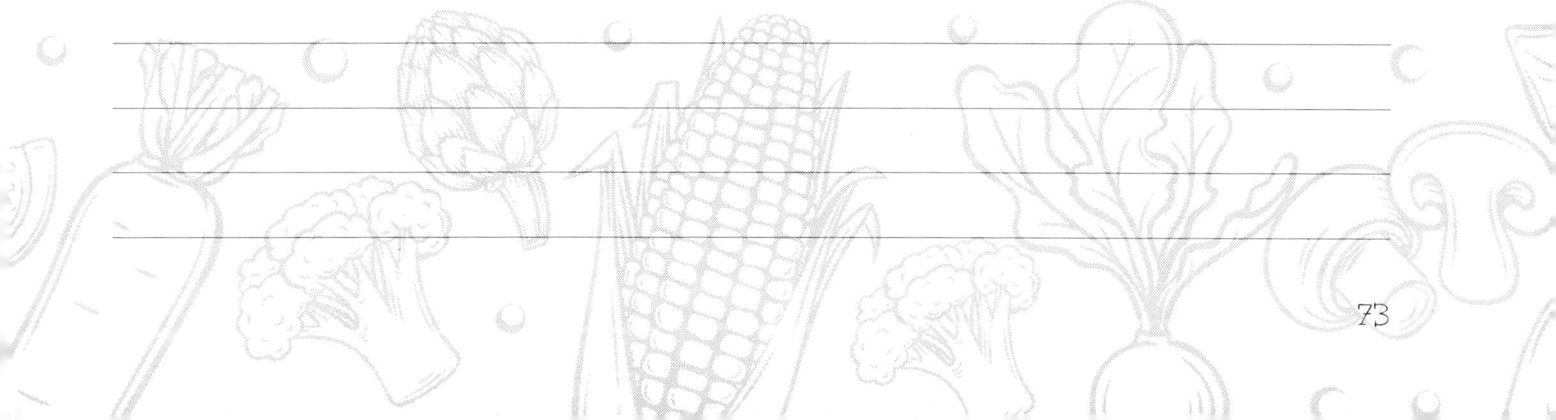

Preparation time: Cook time: Servings:

Ingredients

Method

Preparation time: Cook time: Servings:

Ingredients

Method

Preparation time: Cook time: Servings:

Ingredients

Method

Preparation time: Cook time: Servings:

Ingredients

Method

Preparation time: Cook time: Servings:

Ingredients

Method

Preparation time: Cook time: Servings:

Ingredients

Method

Preparation time: Cook time: Servings:

Ingredients

Method

Preparation time: Cook time: Servings:

Ingredients

Method

Preparation time: Cook time: Servings:

Ingredients

Method

Preparation time: Cook time: Servings:

Ingredients

Method

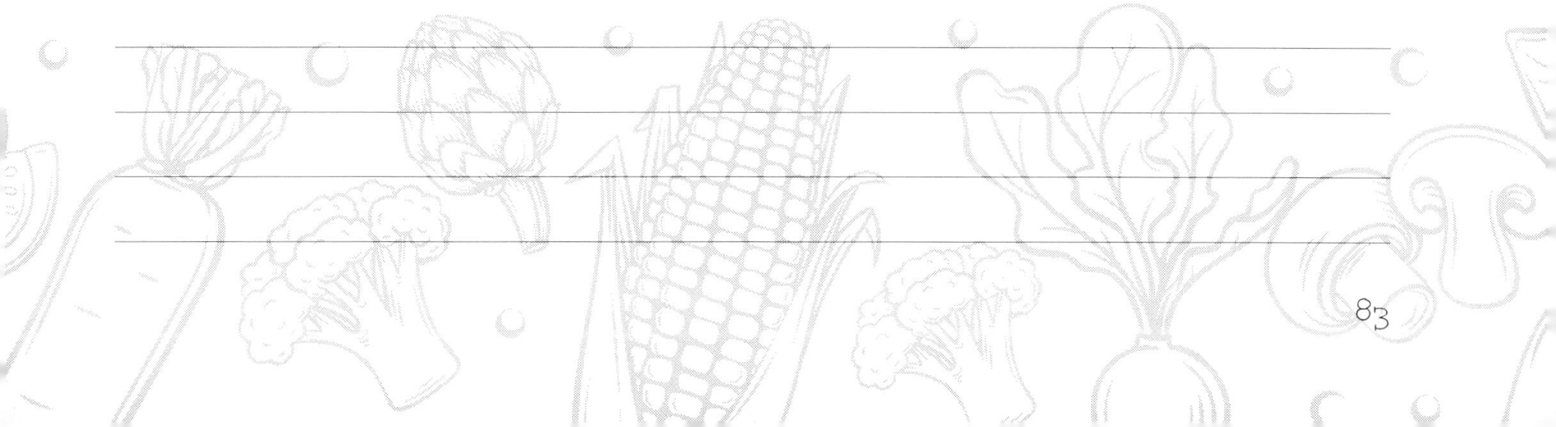

Preparation time: Cook time: Servings:

Ingredients

Method

Preparation time: Cook time: Servings:

Ingredients

Method

Preparation time: Cook time: Servings:

Ingredients

Method

Preparation time: Cook time: Servings:

Ingredients

Method

Preparation time: Cook time: Servings:

Ingredients

Method

Preparation time: Cook time: Servings:

Ingredients

Method

Preparation time: Cook time: Servings:

Ingredients

Method

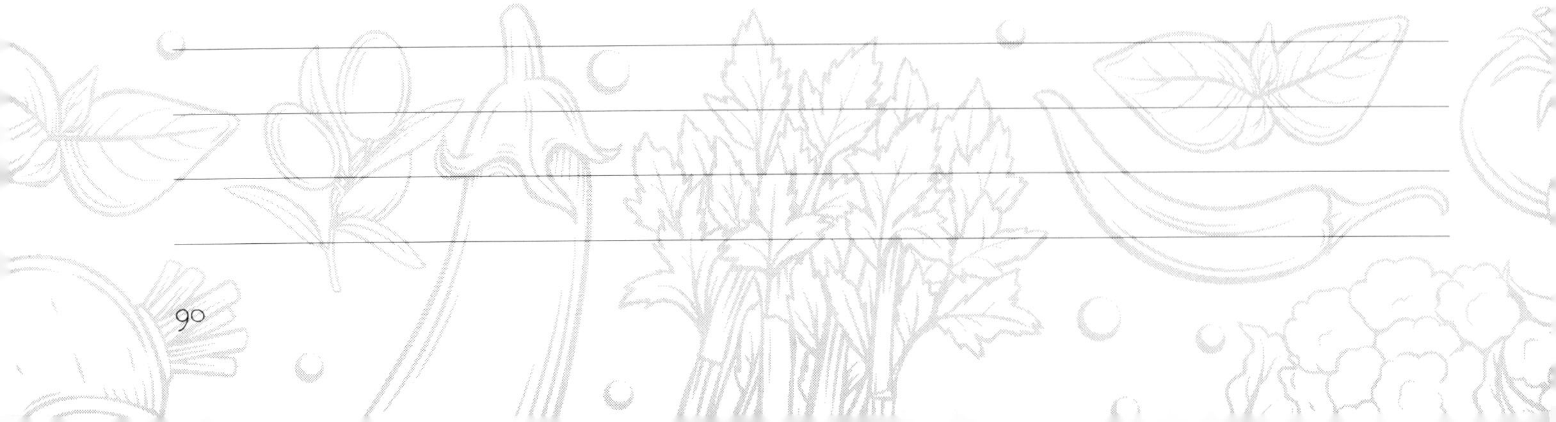

Preparation time: Cook time: Servings:

Ingredients

Method

Preparation time: Cook time: Servings:

Ingredients

Method

Preparation time: Cook time: Servings:

Ingredients

Method

Preparation time: Cook time: Servings:

Ingredients

Method

Preparation time: Cook time: Servings:

Ingredients

Method

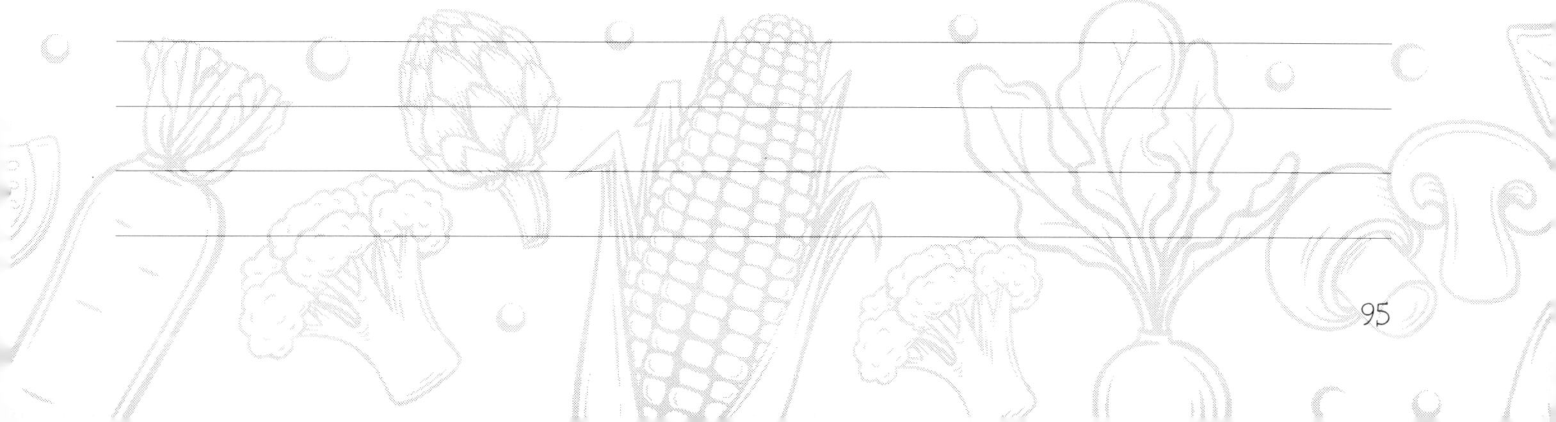

Preparation time: Cook time: Servings:

Ingredients

Method

Preparation time: Cook time: Servings:

Ingredients

Method

Preparation time: Cook time: Servings:

Ingredients

Method

Preparation time: Cook time: Servings:

Ingredients

Method

Preparation time: Cook time: Servings:

Ingredients

Method

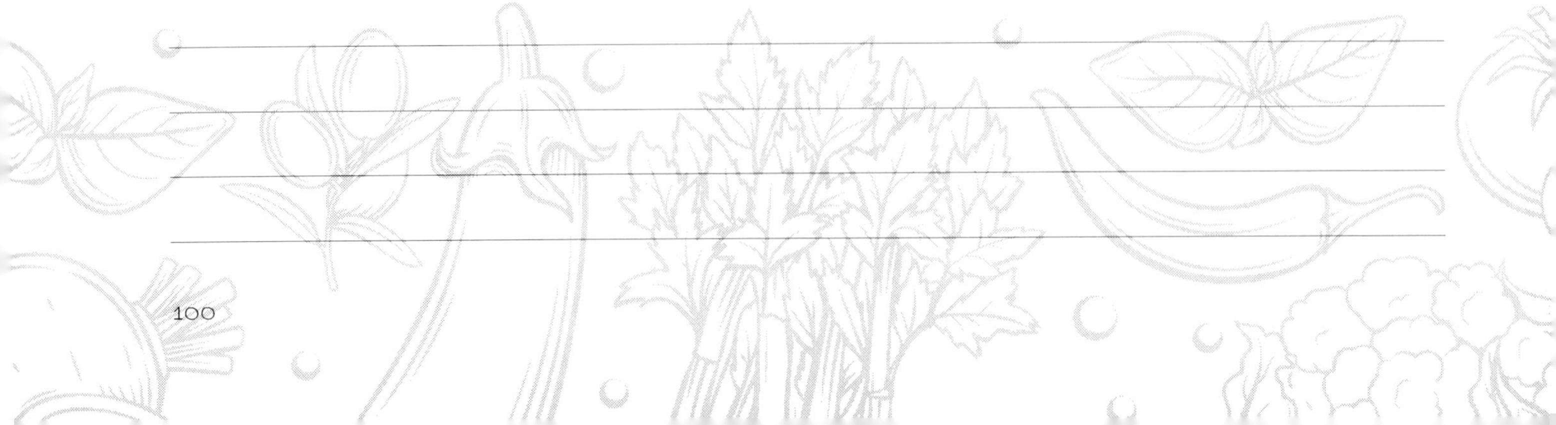

Made in United States
Orlando, FL
07 November 2026

90337526R00059